Chair Yoga for Elderly People with Limited Mobility: Advice and Adjustments to Enhance Mobility, Health, and Posture

Copyright © by Dr Emily k Pitts 2024. All rights reserved.

Disclaimer

The information presented in this article is meant for general educational purposes only and should not be interpreted as medical advice or a substitute for professional consultation, diagnosis, or treatment. Always consult with a healthcare physician before starting any new exercise regimen, particularly if you have current health conditions or concerns. The workouts and adjustments described herein may not be suited for everyone; individual capabilities and limits must be taken into account. The writers and publishers are not responsible for any injury or harm that may arise

from practicing the exercises or following the

advice offered in this article.

About the author

Dr. Emily K. Pitts is an experienced geriatric wellness specialist and a licensed yoga therapist with a passion for encouraging healthy aging. With a Ph.D. in gerontology and over 15 years of experience dealing with elderly populations, Dr. Pitts specializes in establishing adaptive fitness programs that cater to people with limited mobility. Her creative approach to chair yoga has helped numerous elders improve their mobility, health, and posture. In her book, "Chair Yoga for Elderly People with Limited Mobility," Dr. Pitts combines her substantial knowledge and practical experience to provide vital advice and simple yoga adjustments, helping seniors to

enjoy more active and meaningful lives.

Table of contents

- Warm-Up Activities

4. Chair Yoga Pose Fundamentals
- Forward Bend
- Seated Mountain Pose
- Cat-Cow Stretch
- Seated Spinal Twist
- Seated Hip Opener

5. Higher Level Chair Yoga Positions and Adjustments
- Chair Sun Salutations
- Chair Warrior Pose
- Chair Pigeon Pose
- Adjusting Poses for Various Mobility Levels

6. Mindfulness Exercises and Breathing Methods
- Mindfulness via Movement

- Guided Relaxation and Meditation
- Deep Breathing Exercises

7. Developing a Customized Chair Yoga Exercise

- Evaluating personal requirements and capabilities
- Establishing Reasonable Objectives and Making Safe
  Progress Over Time

8. Including Chair Yoga in Everyday Activities

- Quick morning and evening routines
- chair yoga while reading or watching TV
- chair yoga sessions in groups and socializing

9. Case Studies and Success Stories

- Elderly People's Testimonials About How Chair Yoga Improved Their Mobility

Conclusion

- Recap of key points
- Motivation for starting a chair yoga

Introduction

Importance of Chair Yoga for Seniors

Getting older is a normal process that causes a number of changes to occur in the body. These changes frequently result in a reduction in mobility, an increase in stiffness, and an increased likelihood of developing chronic illnesses. Because of these physical restrictions, it might be difficult for many elderly people to participate in traditional types of exercise. Maintaining a regular physical activity routine, on the other hand, is essential for one's general health and prosperity. The practice of chair yoga comes into play at this point. A moderate style of yoga that may be practiced while seated or with the assistance of a chair, chair yoga is a good choice for senior citizens because it can be performed in either position. The purpose of this introduction is to discuss the significance of chair yoga for older citizens, detailing the multiple advantages that it offers and elaborating on the reasons why it is an appropriate form of physical activity for this demographic.

Fostering Physical Health and Wellness

1. Increasing Flexibility and Maintaining Healthy Joints

Our muscles and joints have a tendency to become less flexible as we get older, which can result in stiffness and feelings of discomfort. Chair yoga is a form of yoga that aims to enhance joint flexibility and gently stretch the muscles without putting undue stress on the body. The slow, controlled movements in chair yoga allow a steady increase in range of motion, which can considerably boost general mobility and lessen the risk of accidents.

2. Strengthening Muscles

Maintaining muscle strength is vital for seniors to conduct daily activities independently. Chair yoga contains several positions that target different muscle areas, helping to improve and maintain muscle strength. For instance, positions like seated leg lifts and chair planks engage the core, leg, and arm muscles, offering a comprehensive exercise that enhances functional fitness.

3. Enhancing Balance and Coordination
Falls are a significant issue among seniors, often leading to catastrophic injuries. Chair yoga promotes balance and coordination through precise positions and sequences. By performing balance-enhancing activities in a controlled, seated environment, seniors can enhance their stability and lessen the probability of falling. Poses such as the seated warrior and modified tree pose serve to develop proprioception and overall balance.

4. Boosting Cardiovascular Health
While chair yoga is moderate, it can nevertheless

deliver cardiovascular benefits. Sequences that entail continuous movement, such as seated sun salutations, can help boost the heart rate and enhance circulation. Regular practice of chair yoga can lead to better cardiovascular health, aiding in the prevention of heart disease and other related illnesses.

5. Alleviating Chronic Pain

Chronic pain, particularly in the back, knees, and hips, is a prevalent condition among the elderly. Chair yoga offers a way to manage and reduce pain through mild stretching and strengthening activities. The mindfulness component of yoga also plays a role in pain management by helping patients focus on the breath and build a more positive relationship with their bodies.

Supporting Mental and Emotional Well-Being

1.Reducing Stress and Anxiety

Aging can bring about a number of emotional issues, including stress, worry, and despair. Chair yoga involves breathing exercises and mindfulness practices that help relax the mind and reduce stress. Practices like deep breathing and guided relaxation encourage the release of stress and generate a sense of tranquility and mental clarity.

2. Enhancing Cognitive Function

Regular physical activity, particularly chair yoga, has been demonstrated to enhance cognitive wellness. The mix of movement, coordination, and mindfulness in chair yoga can help boost brain function and improve cognitive capacities such as memory, attention, and problem-solving skills. This is particularly crucial for seniors, as they aim to preserve their mental sharpness and delay the onset of cognitive deterioration.

3. Promoting Social Interaction

Participating in chair yoga courses gives seniors the opportunity to mingle and create connections with others. Social engagement is an important component of emotional well-being, helping to overcome feelings of loneliness and isolation.

Group chair yoga classes offer a friendly environment where elders can share experiences and encourage one another on their wellness journeys.

Facilitating Accessibility and Inclusivity

1.Adaptability for Various Fitness Levels
One of the major advantages of chair yoga is its versatility. Whether a senior is new to exercising or has been active for years, chair yoga can be adapted to meet their unique goals and fitness levels. Modifications and variations of poses ensure that everyone can participate and benefit, regardless of their physical condition or restrictions.

2.Convenience and Ease of Practice
Chair yoga may be practiced practically anywhere, making it a convenient option for elders. Whether at home, in a community center, or in a senior living facility, all that is needed is a sturdy chair and a little bit of room. This convenience eliminates several hurdles to

regular exercise, such as transportation concerns or poor weather.

3.Safe for Individuals with Chronic Conditions
Many seniors live with chronic health concerns such as arthritis, osteoporosis, or cardiovascular disease. Chair yoga is a safe type of exercise that may be customized to fit various circumstances. By focusing on soft movements and avoiding high-impact activities, chair yoga decreases the potential for worsening existing health conditions while still providing major health benefits.

Encouraging a Holistic Approach to Health

1. Integrating Mind, Body, and Spirit
Chair yoga embraces the entire idea of traditional yoga, emphasizing the integration of mind, body, and spirit. This technique allows elders to build a more profound connection with their bodies and creates a sense of general well-being. The practice of chair yoga goes beyond physical exercise, fostering a healthy and

harmonious existence.

2. Empowering Seniors with Self-Care Tools
Chair yoga offers seniors tools to take control of their health and well-being. The skills acquired in chair yoga can be employed throughout the day to manage stress, enhance posture, and reduce tension. This empowerment creates a proactive attitude toward health, encouraging elders to actively participate in their wellness journey.

3.Cultivating a Positive Outlook on Aging
Engaging in chair yoga can help seniors build a more positive view of aging. The practice increases acceptance of the aging process and promotes self-compassion. By focusing on what their bodies can do rather than restrictions, seniors can build a more positive body image and increase their self-esteem.

Chair yoga is a useful practice for seniors,

delivering a number of physical, mental, and emotional advantages. It provides an accessible and adaptive kind of exercise that targets the special demands and challenges of the elderly population. By enhancing flexibility, strength, balance, and cardiovascular health, chair yoga increases total physical well-being. Additionally, its emphasis on mindfulness and social contact helps mental and emotional health. Chair yoga's versatility ensures that it may be done by seniors of all fitness levels and health concerns, making it an inclusive and convenient option.

Incorporating chair yoga into everyday routines encourages seniors to take an active role in their health, creating a holistic approach to well-being. As a mild yet effective type of exercise, chair yoga helps seniors preserve their independence, manage chronic diseases, and improve their quality of life. For these reasons, chair yoga is not just a fitness regimen; it is a gateway to a better, more fulfilling, and more balanced life for seniors.

Chapter 1

Understanding Limited Mobility in the Elderly

Aging is accompanied by different bodily changes that often contribute to decreased mobility. This disorder greatly undermines the quality of life for many elderly adults, affecting their capacity to conduct everyday activities, maintain independence, and engage in social relationships. Understanding the common reasons for limited mobility and its repercussions for daily living and health is vital for designing effective methods to support and promote the well-being of elders.

Common Causes of Limited Mobility

1.Musculoskeletal Disorders
Arthritis: Arthritis, particularly osteoarthritis and rheumatoid arthritis, is a prominent cause of restricted mobility in the elderly. These disorders

induce joint inflammation, discomfort, and stiffness, making movement difficult. Osteoarthritis primarily affects weight-bearing joints, including the knees, hips, and spine, but rheumatoid arthritis can affect various joints throughout the body.

- **Osteoporosis:** Osteoporosis is characterized by weaker bones that are more susceptible to fractures. This condition is frequent among the elderly, especially postmenopausal women. Fractures, particularly of the hip and spine, can dramatically restrict mobility and independence.

2. Neurological Disorders

Stroke: Strokes can result in varied degrees of paralysis or muscle weakness, frequently affecting one side of the body. This can significantly impair mobility and require extensive therapy.

Parkinson's Disease: Parkinson's disease is a progressive neurological illness that affects movement. Symptoms such as tremors, stiffness, and bradykinesia (slowness of movement) can make walking and other motor activities problematic.

Multiple Sclerosis (MS): MS is an autoimmune illness that targets the central nervous system, resulting in mobility impairments owing to muscle weakness, spasms, and coordination deficits.

3. Cardiovascular Conditions

Heart Disease:Conditions including congestive heart failure and coronary artery disease can contribute to reduced physical stamina and endurance, restricting an elderly person's ability to engage in physical activity.
Peripheral Artery Disease (PAD): PAD involves the constriction of blood vessels outside the heart, frequently in the legs, causing pain and cramps during walking or other activities, consequently decreasing mobility.

4. Metabolic Disorders

Diabetes: Diabetes can lead to various issues affecting mobility, such as neuropathy (nerve damage), which causes discomfort and numbness in the extremities, and poor circulation, which can lead to ulcers and infections.

Obesity: Excess body weight puts additional strain on joints and muscles, worsening illnesses like arthritis and increasing the risk of falls and fractures.

5.Respiratory Conditions

Chronic Obstructive Pulmonary Disease (COPD): COPD and other chronic respiratory disorders can impair mobility by producing shortness of breath and exhaustion, making physical activity difficult.

6. Sensory Impairments

eyesight loss:Conditions such as cataracts, glaucoma, and macular degeneration can impair eyesight, making it difficult for the elderly to navigate their surroundings safely and confidently, thereby limiting their mobility.

Hearing Loss: While not directly limiting physical mobility, hearing loss can damage balance and raise the risk of falls.

7. Psychological Factors

Depression: Depression and anxiety can lead to lower motivation for physical activity, resulting in a sedentary lifestyle and a consequent decline in physical capabilities.

Cognitive Decline: Dementia and other cognitive impairments can decrease coordination and balance, increasing the risk of falls and lowering overall mobility.

Consequences for Daily Living and Health

1. Reduced Independence

Limited mobility typically leads to a diminished capacity to complete Activities of Daily Living (ADLs), such as bathing, dressing, eating, and toileting. This loss of freedom can be very disheartening and may entail the need for assistance from caregivers or the shift to assisted living facilities.

2. Increased Risk of Falls

Falls are a big issue for the elderly with limited mobility. Reduced muscle strength, poor balance, and longer reaction times contribute to an increased risk of falls, which can result in fractures, brain injuries, and other significant health issues. The dread of falling can further lower activity levels, producing a vicious cycle of reducing mobility and increasing fall risk.

3. Chronic Pain

Conditions that cause reduced movement, such as arthritis and osteoporosis, are commonly coupled with persistent discomfort. Persistent pain can influence sleep, emotions, and overall quality of life, leading to increased usage of pain drugs, which may have negative effects and interact with other medications.

4. Decreased Physical Fitness

Limited mobility restricts opportunities for physical activity, resulting in deconditioning and muscular atrophy. This decline in physical fitness exacerbates mobility challenges and raises the likelihood of various health problems, such as cardiovascular disease, diabetes, and obesity.

5. Social Isolation

Mobility constraints can make it difficult for the elderly to participate in social activities, resulting in isolation and loneliness. Social isolation is connected with a range of unfavorable health effects, including depression, cognitive impairment, and a higher mortality risk.

6. Mental Health Issues

The psychological impact of reduced movement might be severe. The loss of freedom and the inability to engage in previously enjoyed activities can lead to feelings of frustration, helplessness, and sadness. Anxiety over falls and health decline can further complicate mental health difficulties.

7. Increased Healthcare Utilization

Elderly adults with reduced mobility often require more regular medical care, including doctor visits, physical therapy, and hospitalizations. This increased healthcare consumption can place a huge financial burden on individuals and their families, as well as on the healthcare system.

8. Impact on Caregivers

Limited mobility in the elderly typically demands support from family members or professional caretakers. The duties of caregiving can lead to physical, emotional, and financial strain on caregivers, compromising their health and well-being.

9. Nutritional Challenges

Limited mobility can impair an aging person's ability to shop for groceries, make meals, and eat independently. This can lead to inadequate nutrition, which further weakens the body and exacerbates health difficulties. Malnutrition is a severe concern among the elderly and can lead to reduced immune function, muscle loss, and increased susceptibility to infections.

10. Cognitive Decline

Physical activity is recognized to improve cognitive wellness. Limited mobility generally results in diminished physical exercise, which can contribute to cognitive deterioration. Regular movement helps maintain brain function by boosting blood flow and neuroplasticity. A sedentary lifestyle, therefore, poses dangers to cognitive health, potentially speeding the course of dementia and other cognitive deficits.

Strategies to Mitigate Limited Mobility

Understanding the causes and implications of reduced mobility is the first step in tackling this issue. Several measures can help lessen its impact:

1. Exercise Programs
Tailored exercise regimens that focus on strength, flexibility, and balance can help maintain and enhance mobility. Activities such as chair yoga, water aerobics, and tai chi are particularly useful for the elderly.

2. Physical Therapy

Physical therapists can build individualized plans to treat specific mobility concerns, integrating exercises and strategies to promote movement, reduce pain, and prevent falls.

3. Assistive Devices

The use of assistive equipment, such as walkers, canes, and grab bars, can provide support and stability, making it simpler for the elderly to move around securely and independently.

4. Home Modifications

Simple house improvements, such as ramps, railings, and non-slip flooring, can make a major impact on the safety and accessibility of the living environment for seniors with limited mobility.

5. Medication Management

Proper management of drugs for disorders including arthritis, diabetes, and cardiovascular diseases can help control symptoms that affect mobility. Regular reviews of medication regimens are crucial to avoid side effects that may limit mobility.

6. Nutritional Support

Ensuring that elders have access to good meals and addressing any barriers to optimal nutrition can enhance overall health and mobility. This may comprise meal delivery services, nutritional supplements, or aid with meal preparation.

7. Mental Health Support

Addressing mental health difficulties through therapy, support groups, and pharmaceuticals, when appropriate, can increase motivation and overall well-being, encouraging more active lifestyles.

8. Community Programs

Community programs that offer social activities and physical exercise designed for the elderly can help reduce isolation and promote active engagement in a safe setting.

9. Education and Awareness

Educating elders and their caregivers about the value of physical activity and the options available to retain mobility can empower them to take proactive actions towards improving their health.

Limited mobility in the elderly is a complex issue with varied causes and major effects on everyday functioning and health. Understanding these elements is critical for establishing effective interventions and support systems. By addressing the musculoskeletal, neurological, cardiovascular, metabolic, respiratory, sensory, and psychological elements of reduced mobility, it is feasible to enhance the quality of life for seniors. Implementing focused strategies such as specialized exercise programs, physical therapy, assistive equipment, home modifications, and complete healthcare management can help offset the impact of limited mobility, enabling seniors to preserve their independence, health, and well-being.

Chapter 2

Advantages of Chair Yoga for Elderly People with Low Mobility

Chair yoga is a mild kind of exercise that can be conducted while seated or utilizing a chair for support. It is especially advantageous for elderly people with reduced mobility due to its accessibility and adjustability. Chair yoga has several advantages, from strengthening joint health and flexibility to improving balance, minimizing falls, promoting emotional health, reducing stress, and treating persistent pain and soreness. This complete approach to well-being makes chair yoga a wonderful choice for seniors wishing to maintain or improve their quality of life.

Strengthening Joint Health and Flexibility

As we age, preserving joint health and flexibility becomes increasingly crucial to preserving mobility and freedom. Chair yoga is a safe and effective way for seniors to reach these goals.

1. Joint Health :Gentle Movements, Chair yoga incorporates moderate, regulated motions that help lubricate the joints, reduce stiffness, and enhance range of motion. These movements are particularly good for people with arthritis since they can help lower inflammation and pain.

i. Strengthening Support Muscles: Many chair yoga poses focus on the muscles that support the joints, such as the quadriceps, hamstrings, and muscles surrounding the shoulders and hips. Strengthening these muscles helps to support the joints, minimizing the chance of injury and deterioration.

ii. Increased Circulation: The flowing motions of chair yoga promote blood flow to the joints, providing them with critical nutrients and oxygen. Improved circulation aids in the healing and preservation of joint tissues, enhancing overall joint health.

2. Flexibility: Stretching Exercises:Chair yoga combines a variety of stretching techniques that gradually build flexibility. These stretches are designed to be soft and may be tweaked to suit each individual's abilities, making them accessible for seniors with restricted mobility. Consistent Practice: Regular practice of chair yoga helps to maintain and increase flexibility over time. This constant engagement with stretching activities keeps the muscles and connective tissues from becoming overly tight, which can lead to discomfort and restricted mobility.

Increasing Balance and Reducing Falls

Falls are a big issue for senior adults, often leading to catastrophic injuries and a reduction in independence. Chair yoga can play a key role in strengthening balance and minimizing the risk of falls.

1. Balance Training and Proprioception Improvement: Chair yoga exercises often feature moves that challenge balance and coordination. These exercises strengthen proprioception, the body's ability to detect its position in space. Improved proprioception helps elders react more efficiently to prevent falls.

i. Core Strengthening: Many chair yoga postures utilize the core muscles, which are necessary for maintaining balance and stability. A strong core offers a sturdy basis for all motions, lowering the possibility of losing balance and falling.

ii. Safe Environment: Chair yoga allows elders to practice balance-enhancing activities in a safe atmosphere. The chair provides support, enabling them to do tasks they might not be able to complete standing without assistance.

2. Fall Prevention: Improved Reaction Time: Regular practice of chair yoga can enhance muscle strength and coordination, leading to faster reaction times. This can be vital in preventing falls when faced with unexpected impediments or changes in terrain.

i. Confidence Building: By practicing balance and stability in a controlled environment, seniors can build confidence in their ability to walk safely. This greater confidence can translate to enhanced mobility and a lower risk of falls in routine activities.

ii. Awareness and Mindfulness: Chair yoga increases mindfulness and body awareness, helping seniors be present and focused on their activities. This heightened awareness can help individuals detect and avoid potential hazards, significantly reducing the chance of falling.

Improving Emotional Health and Stress Reduction

Chair yoga is not only excellent for physical health but also plays a key part in promoting mental well-being and lowering stress.

1. Emotional Health;Mood Enhancement: The gentle movements and careful breathing exercises in chair yoga increase the release of endorphins, the body's natural "feel-good" hormones. This can help improve mood and counteract feelings of despair and anxiety, which are frequent among the elderly.

i. Sense of Accomplishment: Completing chair yoga sessions can create a sense of satisfaction and increase self-esteem. This is particularly crucial for elders, who may feel disheartened by physical constraints. The capacity to participate and improve in chair yoga can foster a good view of life.

ii. Social Interaction: Group chair yoga courses give possibilities for social interaction and connection. Building ties with individuals who have similar challenges can provide emotional support and minimize feelings of loneliness and isolation.

2. Stress Reduction: Relaxation Techniques Chair yoga combines relaxation techniques such as deep breathing, guided meditation, and progressive muscle relaxation. These techniques activate the parasympathetic nervous system, encouraging a state of calm and lowering stress levels.

i. Mindfulness and Presence: Chair yoga promotes mindfulness, urging participants to focus on the present moment and their breathing. This mindfulness exercise helps elders separate from worries and negative thoughts, generating a sense of inner calm and tranquility.

ii. Breathing Exercises: Controlled breathing techniques, such as diaphragmatic breathing and alternate nostril breathing, serve to regulate the nervous system and lessen the physiological effects of stress. These approaches can be particularly effective for seniors who endure anxiety or persistent stress.

Relieving Persistent Pain and Soreness

Chronic pain and soreness are typical difficulties among the elderly, sometimes originating from illnesses such as arthritis, fibromyalgia, and past injuries. Chair yoga offers helpful ways for controlling and reducing persistent pain.

1. "Pain Management" and "Gentle Movement" The mild, low-impact movements of chair yoga help to alleviate pain by boosting blood flow, lowering muscle tension, and enhancing joint mobility. These motions can be particularly beneficial for people with chronic pain issues. Endorphin Release: Exercise, particularly chair yoga, encourages the release of endorphins, which are natural pain relievers. The mix of physical movement and relaxation in chair yoga can help to lessen the sense of pain and enhance overall comfort.

Targeted Stretches: Chair yoga involves stretches that target specific parts of the body where pain and discomfort are common. For example, moderate spinal twists can help ease back pain, while seated hip openers can reduce discomfort in the hips and lower back.

2. Soreness Relief; Muscle Relaxation Chair yoga promotes muscle relaxation through a combination of stretching and breathing exercises. Relaxed muscles are less likely to become sore and tight, giving instant and long-term relief from discomfort.

i. Inflammation Reduction: The controlled motions and stretches of chair yoga can help reduce inflammation, a frequent source of discomfort and soreness. Improved circulation and lymphatic flow aid in eliminating inflammatory compounds from the body, aiding healing, and lowering pain.

ii. Holistic Approach: Chair yoga takes a holistic approach to pain management, addressing both the physical and mental components of pain. By mixing mindfulness and relaxation techniques, chair yoga helps seniors manage pain more effectively, minimizing the need for medication and enhancing their overall quality of life.

Chair yoga offers a plethora of advantages for seniors with reduced mobility. By strengthening joint health and flexibility, increasing balance, avoiding falls, improving emotional health, reducing stress, and treating persistent pain and discomfort, chair yoga provides a complete approach to improving well-being. Its mild, adjustable nature makes yoga a great type of exercise for seniors, regardless of their physical limitations.

As a comprehensive practice, chair yoga addresses both the physical and emotional components of health, encouraging a sense of general well-being and improving quality of life. For elderly people seeking a safe, effective, and pleasurable way to stay active and healthy, chair yoga is an excellent tool. By introducing chair yoga into their routine, seniors can maintain their independence, lessen the chance of injury, and experience a higher degree of physical and emotional wellness.

Chapter 3

Introduction to Chair Yoga

Chair yoga is an adaptation of traditional yoga practices that allows participants to perform yoga poses while seated or using a chair for support. This kind of yoga is particularly good for older adults, people with disabilities, or those recuperating from injuries, as it gives a gentle yet effective technique to enhance physical fitness, flexibility, and mental well-being without the need for advanced strength or balance.

Chair yoga offers a holistic approach to health, embracing physical, mental, and emotional aspects. It offers a variety of positions and exercises that may be readily adapted to meet individual requirements and restrictions. By incorporating breathing methods, mindfulness, and relaxation exercises, chair yoga provides a holistic wellness program that can be done by people of various fitness levels.

Selecting the Appropriate Chair and Equipment

Choosing the correct chair and equipment is vital for a safe and effective chair yoga practice. Here are some guidelines to help you select the suitable gear:

1. The Chair; Stability; Ensure the chair is stable and strong. It should not bend or be sliding on the floor. Chairs with rubber grips on the feet are great as they provide added stability.

i.Back Support: A chair with a straight back is recommended, as it gives appropriate support for the spine. Avoid seats with wheels or those that recline.

ii. Height: The chair should be at an acceptable height so that when you sit, your feet are flat on the floor and your knees are at a right angle. This alignment helps maintain normal posture and saves pressure on the joints.

 iii. Seat Surface:The seat should be firm and flat, offering a secure base for sitting. Avoid overly padded or soft seats that might impact balance and posture.

2. Additional Equipment :Yoga Mat: Place a yoga mat under the chair to prevent it from slipping and to offer a soft platform for any standing or floor activities.

i. Blocks and Straps: Yoga blocks and straps can be used to modify poses and give extra support. They are especially effective for people with limited flexibility or range of motion.

ii. Blankets and Cushions: These can be utilized for increased comfort and support during seated poses. A folded blanket can also function as a cushion for the lower back or knees.

Safety Procedures and Instructions

Safety is crucial when practicing chair yoga, especially for people with limited mobility or health concerns. Here are some crucial safety practices and instructions:

1. Consult with a Healthcare Professional: Before beginning any new fitness program, including chair yoga, consult with a healthcare provider to confirm it is safe for you. This is particularly critical for people with chronic diseases, recent surgeries, or serious health issues.

2. Warm-Up; Always start with a warm-up to prepare your body for the workouts. Gentle motions and stretches promote blood flow to the muscles and lessen the risk of injury.

3. Listen to Your Body: Pay attention to how your body feels during each pose. If you develop pain, dizziness, or shortness of breath, stop

immediately and rest. Modify positions as needed to match your comfort level and abilities.

4. Maintain Proper Posture: Focus on maintaining proper alignment throughout the practice. Sit up straight with your back supported by the chair, feet flat on the floor, and shoulders relaxed. This posture helps prevent strain and damage.

5. Breathe Mindfully: Coordinate your motions with your breath. Inhale deeply via the nose and exhale fully through the mouth. Mindful breathing helps oxygenate your muscles and promotes calm.

6. Use Supportive Equipment: Utilize blocks, straps, and cushions to modify poses and provide additional support. These props can help you

attain perfect alignment and lessen the danger of strain or damage.

7. Move Slowly and Gently: Perform each action slowly and gently. Avoid jerky or fast moves that can lead to harm. Gradually expand the range of motion as your body becomes more acclimated to the activities.

8. Hydrate: Keep a water bottle available and stay hydrated throughout the practice. Proper hydration is vital for general health and helps sustain muscle function.

9. Cool Down: End each session with a cool-down period, including moderate stretches and relaxation techniques. This helps your body shift back to a resting state and reduces muscle stiffness.

Warm-Up Activities

A proper warm-up is crucial to preparing the body for chair yoga practice. Here are some great warm-up activities to get started:

1. "Seated Marching: Sit up straight with your feet flat on the floor.

Lift one leg toward your chest while keeping your core engaged.

Lower your foot back to the floor and repeat with the opposite leg.

Continue alternating legs for 1-2 minutes to enhance heart rate and circulation.

2. Ankle and Wrist Circles; Sit comfortably with your feet flat on the floor.

Lift one foot slightly off the ground and rotate your ankle in a circular manner, both clockwise and counterclockwise, for 10–15 seconds per way.

Repeat with the opposite ankle.

Extend your arms in front of you and rotate your wrists in circular motions, both clockwise and counterclockwise, for 10–15 seconds per way.

3. Shoulder Rolls: Sit up straight with your feet flat on the floor and arms relaxed at your sides.

Lift your shoulders toward your ears, then roll them back and down in a circular motion.

Repeat this movement for 10–15 seconds, then reverse the direction and roll your shoulders forward.

4. Neck Stretches: Sit comfortably with your feet flat on the floor and your back straight.

Slowly tilt your head to the right, bringing your ear toward your shoulder. Hold for 10–15 seconds, then return to the center.

Repeat on the left side.

Gently swivel your head to look over your right shoulder, hold for 10–15 seconds, then return to center. Repeat on the left side.

5. Seated Cat-Cow Stretch: Sit with your feet flat on the floor and hands resting on your knees.

Inhale and arch your back, elevating your chest and looking up (Cow Pose).

Exhale and curve your spine, tucking your chin to your chest (cat pose).

Continue moving between these two postures with your breath for 1-2 minutes to warm up your spine and back muscles.

6. Arm Raises: Sit with your feet flat on the floor and your back straight.

After letting out a breath, return your arms to your sides.

Repeat this movement 5–10 times, coordinating with your breath.

7. Seated Twist: Sit with your feet flat on the floor and your back straight.

Position your right hand behind your chair and your left hand on your right thigh.

Inhale and stretch your spine, then exhale and slowly twist your torso to the right, gazing over your right shoulder.

Hold for 10–15 seconds, then return to the center.

Repeat on the left side.

8. Toe Taps : Sit with your feet flat on the floor and your back straight.

Lift your toes while maintaining your heels on the ground, then lower them back down.

Continue this exercise for 1-2 minutes to warm up your lower legs and feet.

9. Finger Stretches: Extend your arms in front of you with your palms facing down.

Spread your fingers wide apart, then close them into a fist.

Repeat this action 10–15 times to warm up your hands and fingers.

10. Breathing Exercises: Sit comfortably with your feet flat on the floor and your back straight.

Close your eyes and take several deep breaths, inhaling through your nose and exhaling through your mouth.

Focus on your breath and strive to extend each inhale and exhale.

Continue this breathing technique for 1-2 minutes to relax your thoughts and prepare for the practice.

Chair yoga offers a safe and accessible alternative for senior adults with reduced mobility to enjoy the benefits of yoga. By selecting the appropriate chair and equipment, sticking to safety precautions, and implementing effective warm-up exercises, seniors can enhance their physical, mental, and emotional well-being through regular chair yoga practice.

This gentle form of exercise helps improve joint health, flexibility, balance, emotional health, and overall quality of life, making it an excellent complement to any wellness program for people with limited mobility.

Chapter 4

Chair Yoga Pose Fundamentals

Chair yoga is a versatile and accessible style of yoga that may be performed while seated or using a chair for support. This strategy makes yoga more inclusive for older adults, people with impairments, or anyone with movement constraints. Understanding the fundamental poses of chair yoga is vital for building a safe and effective practice. Here, we will examine five fundamental chair yoga poses: forward bend, seated mountain pose, cat-cow stretch, seated spinal twist, and seated hip opener.

Forward Bend

The forward bend stance is wonderful for extending the back, hamstrings, and calves. It also helps to quiet the mind and relieve tension.

1. Positioning: Sit on the edge of the chair with your feet flat on the floor, hip-width apart.
Ensure your back is straight and your hands rest on your thighs.

2. Execution: Inhale deeply, stretching your spine.
As you exhale, hinge at your hips and progressively bend forward, maintaining your back straight.
Allow your arms to dangle down toward the floor, or if you are more flexible, you can reach for your feet or ankles.
Let your head and neck relax, and take a few deep breaths in this position.

3. Modification: If you have lower back

concerns or limited flexibility, lay your hands on your thighs and bend only as far as is comfortable.

Use a cushion or yoga block to rest your hands on if you cannot reach the floor.

4. Benefits: Stretches the back, hamstrings, and calves.

improves flexibility in the spine and hips.

reduces tension and promotes relaxation.

enhances digestion by gently massaging abdominal organs.

Seated Mountain Pose

Seated Mountain Pose is a basic position that promotes good alignment and balance. It acts as a starting point for various chair yoga positions and helps improve posture.

1. Positioning: Sit up straight on the chair with your feet flat on the floor and your knees at a 90-degree angle.

Place your hands on your thighs or let them hang

freely at your sides.
Ensure your shoulders are relaxed and your chin is parallel to the floor.

2. Execution: Inhale deeply, feeling your spine stretch and your chest lift.
Engage your core muscles and keep your back straight.
Imagine a cord tugging the top of your head toward the ceiling, elongating your neck.
Hold this pose for several breaths, maintaining a sense of stability and balance.

3. Modification: If you have difficulties sitting upright, use a cushion or rolled-up towel behind your lower back for additional support.
For increased support, grip onto the sides of the chair.

4. Benefits: Promotes good posture and alignment.
strengthens the core muscles.
enhances balance and stability.
increases awareness of body placement.

Cat-Cow Stretch

The cat-cow stretch is a dynamic movement that develops flexibility in the spine and helps to reduce stress in the back and neck.

1. Positioning: Sit on the edge of the chair with your feet flat on the floor, hip-width apart.
Place your hands on your knees or thighs.

2. Execution: Inhale and arch your back, elevating your chest, and looking up (Cow Pose).
Exhale and circle your back, lowering your chin to your chest and bringing your belly button toward your spine (cat pose).
Continue moving between these two postures, matching your movements with your breath.
Repeat for 5–10 breaths, feeling the stretch along your spine.

3. Modification: If you have limited mobility in your back or neck, execute smaller, more

controlled movements.
Focus on the breath and soft movement rather than the range of motion.

4. Benefits: Increases flexibility and mobility in the spine.
relieves tension and stress in the back and neck.
improves posture and alignment.
enhances coordination and body awareness.

Seated Spinal Twist

The seated spinal twist is a gentle twisting pose that helps to enhance spinal flexibility and digestion while alleviating stress in the back.

1. Positioning: Sit up straight on the chair with your feet flat on the floor and your knees at a 90-degree angle.
Place your hands on your thighs.

2. Execution: Inhale deeply, stretching your spine.
As you exhale, slowly twist your torso to the

right, placing your left hand on your right knee and your right hand on the back of the chair for support.
Hold the twist for several breaths, keeping your spine long and your shoulders relaxed.
Inhale to return to the center, then repeat the twist on the left side.

3. Modification: If you have limited mobility in your spine, execute a smaller twist and avoid pushing yourself beyond your comfort zone.
Make use of a cushion or towel to support your lower back if needed.

4. Benefits: Improves spinal flexibility and rotation.
enhances digestion by massaging the abdominal organs.
relieves stiffness in the back and shoulders.
promotes cleansing and circulation.

Seated Hip Opener

The seated hip opener is a great position for

strengthening flexibility in the hips and alleviating tension in the lower back and legs.

1. Positioning: Sit on the edge of the chair with your feet flat on the floor, hip-width apart.
Place your hands on your thighs.

2. Execution: Inhale deeply, stretching your spine.
As you exhale, elevate your right foot and lay your right ankle on your left knee, producing a figure-four formation.
Softly press down on your right knee to make a deep stretch on your hip.
Hold this position for several breaths, keeping your back straight and your shoulders relaxed.
Inhale to return to the beginning position, then repeat the stretch with your left leg.

3. Modification: If placing your ankle on your knee is too tough, place your foot on the opposite thigh or use a yoga strap to aid with the stretch.
Support your lower back with a cushion or

rolled-up towel if needed.

4. Benefits: Increases flexibility in the hips and lower back.
relieves tension and stiffness in the hips and legs.
improves circulation in the lower body.
enhances general mobility and posture.

Chair yoga provides a safe, accessible, and effective approach for people with restricted mobility to experience the benefits of yoga. By studying and practicing foundational poses such as the Forward Bend, Seated Mountain Pose, Cat-Cow Stretch, Seated Spinal Twist, and Seated Hip Opener, practitioners can increase their physical fitness, flexibility, and mental well-being. Each posture offers unique advantages and may be tweaked to meet individual needs, making chair yoga a versatile and inclusive practice.

Incorporating these essential poses into a daily chair yoga exercise can lead to considerable benefits for overall health and quality of life. The gentle motions and attentive breathing associated with chair yoga promote relaxation, reduce tension, and boost emotional well-being. Additionally, the physical benefits of enhanced flexibility, improved posture, and reduced tension contribute to a more active and independent lifestyle.

Whether performed in a group context or independently, chair yoga provides a supportive and adaptive alternative for people of all fitness levels to engage in physical activity and boost their overall well-being. By embracing the ideas and practices of chair yoga, seniors and those with mobility issues can enjoy a holistic approach to health and wellness that supports the body, mind, and spirit.

Chapter 5

Higher Level Chair Yoga Positions and Adjustments

Chair yoga provides an accessible entrance point to yoga for people with mobility problems. However, it also offers complex poses that can challenge and benefit even those with higher mobility skills. This article discusses higher-level chair yoga positions, including Chair Sun Salutations, Chair Warrior Pose, and Chair Pigeon Pose, and includes information on adapting these poses for varied mobility levels.

Chair Sun Salutations

Chair Sun Salutations are a variation of the conventional Sun Salutation sequence, designed to be performed while seated. This sequence is ideal for warming up the body, improving circulation, and promoting flexibility and strength.

1.Mountain Pose (Tadasana) Starting Position:Sit up straight with your feet flat on the floor, hip-width apart. Place your hands on your thighs.
Action:Inhale and raise your arms upward, palms facing each other. Engage your core and stretch your spine.

2. Forward Bend (Uttanasana)Starting Position:From Mountain Pose, exhale and hinge at your hips, pulling your torso forward. Allow your arms to hang down toward the floor or rest them on your thighs.
Action: Keep your back straight and relax your neck. Take a few deep breaths in this position.

3. Halfway pull (Ardha Uttanasana) Starting Position: From the forward bend, inhale and pull your torso halfway up, resting your hands on your knees or thighs for support.

Action: Keep your back flat and your attention forward. Engage your core to support your lower back.

4. Seated Mountain Pose (Tadasana) Starting Position: From the halfway lift, inhale and return to the starting position, extending your arms high.
Action:Lengthen your spine and engage your core.

5. Seated Backbend (Ardha Chakrasana) Starting Position: From Seated Mountain Pose, exhale and bring your hands to the back of your chair, or place them on your lower back for support.
Action: Inhale and gradually arch your back, elevating your chest toward the ceiling. Keep your neck long and avoid pinching your lower back.

6. Repeat pattern: repeat the pattern multiple times, matching your motions with your breath. This helps to increase strength, flexibility, and coordination.

Chair Warrior Pose

Chair Warrior Pose adapts the conventional Warrior Pose to a sitting posture, delivering the benefits of strength and stability without requiring standing balance.

1. Chair Warrior I (Virabhadrasana I) Starting Position: Sit sideways on the chair with your right side toward the chair's back. Your right leg should be bent at a 90-degree angle with the knee directly over the ankle and your left leg extended straight behind you.

Action:Inhale and raise your arms upward, palms facing each other. Keep your torso looking forward and your hips squared.

Modification: If extending the back leg is difficult, you can keep it bent and place the toes on the floor for support.

2. Chair Warrior II (Virabhadrasana II) Starting Position: From Chair Warrior I, lower your arms to shoulder height, stretching them out to the sides with palms facing down.

Action: Turn your head to glance over your right hand. Ensure your torso remains upright and your hips stay squared.
Modification:If extending the arms is problematic, keep your hands on your hips or use a yoga strap to help with alignment.

3. Chair Reverse Warrior (Viparita Virabhadrasana) Starting Position: From Chair Warrior II, lower your left hand to the back of the chair or your left thigh.

Action: Inhale and reach your right arm aloft, stretching the right side of your body. Look up

towards your right hand, keeping your chest open.
Modification: If reaching overhead is problematic, place your right hand on your shoulder and perform a moderate side bend.

4. Repeat on the Other Side: After completing the sequence on one side, turn to the other side of the chair and repeat the poses with your left leg front.

Chair Pigeon Pose

Chair Pigeon Pose is a version of the conventional Pigeon Pose that targets the hips, glutes, and lower back. This position is beneficial for reducing tension and enhancing flexibility in the hips.

1. Starting Position; Positioning: Sit on the edge of the chair with your feet flat on the floor, hip-width apart. Place your hands on your thighs.

Action: Lift your right foot and lay your right ankle on your left knee, producing a figure-four shape. Flex your right foot to protect your knee.

2. Forward Fold:Positioning: Inhale and stretch your spine.

Action: As you exhale, hinge at your hips and lean forward, maintaining your back straight. Rest your hands on your thighs or on the floor if you can.
Modification: If bending forward is too intense, stay upright and softly press down on your right knee with your hand to deepen the stretch.

3. Hold and breathe. Positioning: Maintain the forward fold or upright position.
Action: Take several deep breaths, feeling the stretch in your right hip and glute. Relax into the pose and avoid forcing the stretch.

Modification:If placing the ankle on the knee is too tough, lay the right foot on the left thigh or use a yoga strap to help with the stretch.

4. Switch sides: After holding the posture for several breaths, release and repeat on the other side with your left ankle on your right knee.

Adjusting Poses for Various Mobility Levels

Chair yoga may be tailored to fit varying mobility levels, ensuring that everyone can participate safely and successfully. Here are some guidelines for altering poses to fit differing abilities:

1. Use Supportive Props (Blocks and Straps): Yoga blocks and straps can provide additional support and help adjust positions. For example, use a block beneath your hands in Forward Bend or a strap to help reach your feet in Seated Pigeon Pose.

Cushions and Towels: Place a pillow or rolled-up towel under your lower back for extra support during seated positions. You can also place a cushion beneath your hips in pigeon pose to make the stretch more accessible.

2. Modify Range of Motion: Smaller Movements: For people with limited flexibility or mobility, conduct smaller, controlled movements. For example, in the Cat-Cow Stretch, emphasis is placed on mild tilting of the pelvis rather than a full spinal movement.
Partial Poses: Instead of fully extending into a stance, alter the position to a partial pose. In Chair Warrior, maintain the rear leg bent and the toes on the floor if extending the leg fully is tough.

3. Seated Adjustments : Stay Seated:For people with balance difficulties or significant mobility restrictions, remain totally seated. For example, execute the seated mountain pose with hands resting on thighs rather than extending aloft.
Supportive Chair Use:Use the back of the chair for support during twisting postures or rest hands on the chair's seat for balance during

forward bending.

4. Focus on Breath and Alignment: Breath Coordination:Emphasize coordinating movements with breath, which helps maintain a safe and successful practice. Encourage deep, deliberate breathing to enhance relaxation and attention.
Good Alignment: Ensure good alignment in all poses to prevent strain and injury. For example, in Seated Mountain Pose, keep the back straight, feet flat on the floor, and shoulders relaxed.

5. Gradual Progression: Start Slowly: Begin with simple postures and progressively progress to more advanced variants as strength and flexibility increase. This method helps improve confidence and decreases the danger of damage.
Individual Pace: Encourage individuals to walk at their own pace, respecting their bodies's boundaries. Remind them that it's good to take pauses and adjust poses as required.

Conclusion

Chair yoga offers a dynamic and inclusive alternative for people with varied levels of mobility to enjoy the benefits of yoga. Higher-level chair yoga positions, such as Chair Sun Salutations, Chair Warrior Pose, and Chair Pigeon Pose, provide more advanced alternatives for those wishing to deepen their practice. By adapting poses for different mobility abilities and using supportive props, everyone may participate safely and successfully.

The key to a successful chair yoga practice is to prioritize safety, appropriate alignment, and conscious breathing. Whether you're a beginner or an experienced yogi, chair yoga can promote physical fitness, flexibility, and mental well-being. Embrace the adaptability of chair yoga and discover the benefits of these higher-level poses to build a holistic and fulfilling practice.

Chapter 6

Mindfulness Exercises and Breathing Methods

The practice of mindfulness, which has its origins in ancient traditions, has recently gained a great deal of appeal in modern culture as a result of the numerous benefits it has been shown to have for mental, emotional, and physical well-being. The practice of mindfulness is centered on a variety of breathing techniques and exercises that assist individuals in becoming more present and in tune with their thoughts, feelings, and the sensations that occur within their bodies. Movement, guided relaxation and meditation, and deep breathing exercises are some of the ways that this article examines the world of mindfulness. It also provides some practical insights into how these practices might be applied to daily life to improve general health.

Mindfulness via Physical Activity

Utilizing mindful awareness in conjunction with physical exercise is what is meant by the term "mindfulness via movement." A more profound connection between the mind and the body can be developed through the practice of mindfulness, which places an emphasis on being present in the moment and paying attention to the sensations, movements, and breath of the body. Movement-based practices such as yoga, tai chi, and mindful walking are examples of common types of mindfulness through movement.

1. Yoga: Yoga is a practice that blends meditation, physical postures, and control of the breath. The practice teaches participants to concentrate on their breathing as well as the sensations that occur within their bodies as they move through a variety of poses. Practitioners are able to build a heightened state of

awareness and inner calm by doing each exercise with careful focus, which allows them to achieve their personal goals. For example, during a sun salutation sequence, one may focus on the stretch in the muscles, the stability of the posture, and the rhythm of the breath, anchoring attention to the present moment.

2. Tai Chi: Tai Chi is a style of martial art recognized for its calm, flowing movements and intense attention to breath and body awareness. Practicing Tai Chi comprises a series of movements executed in a calm, beautiful manner, each flowing into the next without stopping. This fluid movement, paired with deep, controlled breathing, assists in boosting focus, lowering stress, and producing a sense of serenity. Practitioners often remark on a sensation of meditative peace that develops from the continuous, attentive movement.

3. Mindful Walking: Mindful walking converts

an everyday activity into a meditation. By walking slowly and paying close attention to each step, the feelings in the feet, and the surrounding surroundings, individuals can build a state of mindfulness. The goal is to walk with intention, focusing on the movement of the legs, the shift in balance, and the contact of the feet with the ground. This technique can be extremely grounding, helping people feel more connected to the present moment and their physical bodies.

Guided Relaxation and Meditation

Guided relaxation and meditation are important strategies for obtaining mental clarity, emotional balance, and physical relaxation. These techniques entail following spoken instructions that move the mind and body into a state of deep relaxation and mindfulness.

1. Body Scan Meditation: In body scan meditation, individuals are instructed to focus on different regions of their body, from the toes to

the head, recognizing any sensations, stress, or discomfort. This technique aids in relieving physical tension and creates a sense of bodily awareness. The body scan can be particularly useful for those who battle with anxiety or chronic pain, as it develops a non-judgmental awareness of physical sensations, increasing relaxation and acceptance.

2. Progressive Muscle Relaxation (PMR): PMR involves tensing and then gently relaxing distinct muscle groups in the body. A typical session starts with the toes and continues upwards to the head, with the guide urging participants to tense each muscle area for a few seconds before releasing. This practice aids in detecting regions of tension and actively letting go of stress, promoting a profound sense of relaxation and tranquility.

3. Guided Imagery: Guided imagery involves envisioning tranquil and serene scenes or experiences. The guide guides individuals through a narrative that inspires sensory

experiences, such as the sound of waves, the warmth of the sun, or the smell of a forest. This technique leverages the power of the imagination to generate a state of deep relaxation and emotional tranquility. Guided imagery can be particularly effective for lowering stress and anxiety, increasing mood, and promoting overall well-being.

4. Mindfulness Meditation: In mindfulness meditation, individuals are instructed to focus on their breath, thoughts, and feelings without judgment. The guide delivers gentle reminders to bring attention back to the present moment whenever the mind wanders. This technique aids in establishing a state of attentive awareness, where individuals may examine their thoughts and feelings without becoming caught up in them. Regular practice of mindfulness meditation has been demonstrated to reduce stress, promote emotional regulation, and improve general mental health.

Deep Breathing Exercises

Breathing is a vital part of mindfulness and relaxation. Deep breathing exercises can help in soothing the nervous system, lowering tension, and enhancing mental clarity. These exercises focus on managing the breath to generate a sense of calm and mindfulness.

1. Diaphragmatic Breathing: Also known as belly breathing, diaphragmatic breathing includes inhaling deeply into the diaphragm rather than shallowly into the chest. To practice this, one can place a hand on the belly and another on the chest, breathing deeply through the nose so that the belly rises, and expelling slowly through the mouth. This approach promotes the oxygen exchange in the body, increasing relaxation and reducing stress levels.

2. 4-7-8 Breathing: The 4-7-8 technique, developed by Dr. Andrew Weil, is a simple yet powerful strategy for relaxation. It entails inhaling through the nose for a count of four, holding the breath for a count of seven, and then

exhaling entirely through the mouth for a count of eight. This rhythm aids in slowing down the breath, soothing the mind, and generating a sense of relaxation. Regular practice of 4-7-8 breathing can help in reducing anxiety, improving sleep, and promoting general emotional well-being.

3. Box Breathing: Also known as square breathing, box breathing involves inhaling, holding, exhaling, and holding the breath again, each for an equal count, often four. This strategy is often utilized by sports and military personnel to boost attention and minimize stress. To practice box breathing, one can visualize breathing along the edges of a square, inhaling for four counts, holding for four, exhaling for four, and holding again for four. This approach aids in controlling the breath, soothing the nervous system, and enhancing concentration.

4. Alternate Nostril Breathing: Alternate nostril breathing, or Nadi Shodhana, is a yogic practice that involves breathing through one nostril at a

time. This procedure is said to balance the left and right hemispheres of the brain, enhancing mental clarity and emotional harmony. To practice, one can use the thumb to close the right nostril and inhale through the left, then close the left nostril with the ring finger, exhale through the right, inhale through the right, and finally exhale through the left. This cycle is repeated multiple times, generating a sense of peace and equilibrium.

Integrating Mindfulness and Breathing into Daily Life

Incorporating mindfulness exercises and breathing strategies into daily life can dramatically boost overall well-being. Here are some practical strategies for integrating these practices into everyday routines:

1. Start Small: Begin with brief sessions of mindfulness or deep breathing exercises, gradually increasing the duration as you feel

more comfortable with the practice. Even a few minutes of mindful breathing or guided relaxation can have a significant influence.

2. Create a Routine: Establish a regular practice time, whether it's first thing in the morning, during a lunch break, or before bedtime. Consistency assists in making mindfulness a habit and reaping its long-term benefits.

3. Use technology: utilize mindfulness and meditation apps that offer guided sessions, reminders, and progress tracking. These tools can give your practice direction and assistance.

4. Incorporate mindfulness into daily tasks: practice mindfulness during routine tasks such as eating, walking, or commuting. Pay attention to the sensations, sights, and sounds around you, bringing a focused awareness to each moment.

5.Join a Group: Consider joining a mindfulness or meditation group, either in-person or online. Group practice can provide encouragement, support, and a sense of community.

6. Be patient and compassionate. Remember that mindfulness is a journey, not a destination. Be patient with yourself and exercise self-compassion, especially on days when the mind feels particularly restless.

mindfulness exercises and breathing practices offer a doorway to better self-awareness, emotional regulation, and overall well-being. By incorporating mindfulness via movement, guided relaxation and meditation, and deep breathing exercises into their daily lives, individuals can create a sense of presence and tranquility, boosting their quality of life and resilience in the face of life's obstacles.

Chapter 7

Developing a Customized Chair Yoga Exercise

Chair yoga is a mild type of yoga that can be performed while seated, making it accessible to people with varied levels of mobility and fitness. It is particularly good for seniors, people with impairments, or those healing from trauma. Developing a customized chair yoga fitness regimen requires evaluating personal requirements and capabilities, establishing appropriate objectives, and ensuring safe growth over time. This comprehensive guide will help you establish a tailored chair yoga practice that matches your specific needs and improves your general well-being.

Evaluating Personal Requirements and Capabilities

Before commencing a chair yoga practice, it is

necessary to analyze your physical condition, medical history, and personal goals. This examination will help you help you personalize the exercises to your specific needs and ensure they are safe and effective.

Physical Condition and Mobility

1. Assessing Range of Motion: Begin by analyzing your existing range of motion in various joints, suchas your as your shoulders, hips, knees, and spine. This assessment can be done with basic movements such as such as arm circles, leg lifts, and moderate twists. Understanding your limitations will aid in selecting appropriate activities that do not strain your joints.

2. Identifying Pain Points: Take note of any areas where you experience pain or discomfort. These could be chronic disorders like arthritis or acute ailments such as muscle discomfort. It is crucial to avoid workouts that increase these pain sites and to focus on movements that bring

relief and encourage recovery.

3. Strength and Endurance Levels: Evaluate your muscle strength and cardiovascular endurance. This can be done by doing by doing basic tests like standing up from a seated position without using your hands or walking a short distance. Knowing your strength and endurance levels will aid in building a chair yoga routine that is tough yet feasible.

Medical History and Conditions

1. Consulting with a Healthcare ExpertExpert: If you have any chronic medical concerns, recent injuries, or surgeries, it is important to check with a healthcare expert before commencing a chair yoga practice. They can provide recommendations on which moves are safe and which should be avoided.

2. Understanding Medical Limitations: Be aware of any medical issues that may impair your ability to execute specific workouts. For

example, peoplepeople with hypertension should avoid poses that entail inversions or extreme bending. Knowing these restrictions will help in personalizing the technique to ensure safety.

Personal Goals and Preferences

1. Setting Clear Goals: Define what you aim to achieve with your chair yoga practice. Your goals may include improving flexibility, building strength, lowering stress, or enhancing overall well-being. Clear goals will determine the selection of workouts and the organization of your regimen.

2. Identifying Preferences: Consider your particular preferences forfor the type and intensity of exercises. Some folks may prefer a more meditative approach focused on breathwork and relaxation, while others may seek a more dynamic practice that involves strength-building activities. Tailoring the practice to your tastes will enhance motivation and satisfaction.

Establishing Reasonable Objectives and Making Safe Progress Over Time

Once you have analyzed your specific requirements and capabilities, the next stage is to identify reasonable targets and construct a strategy for safe progress. This requires setting realistic goals, designing a balanced routine, and reviewing your progress to ensure continual growth.

Setting realistic and achievable goals

1. Short-term Goals: Start with short-term goals that can be achieved within a few weeks. These could include increasing the duration of your practice, mastering specific postures, or improving flexibility in certain areas. Short-term goals provide a sense of accomplishment andan incentive an incentive to continue.

2. Long-term Goals: Set long-term goals that represent your entire vision for your chair yoga

practice. These can include obtaining more overall flexibility, improving posture, or keeping a regular practice for overall health. Long-term goals provide direction and purpose, helping you stay devoted to your practice.

3. SMART Goals: Ensure your goals are specificspecific, measurable, achievable, relevant, and time-bound. For example, instead of creating a generic goal like "improve flexibility," set a SMART goal such as "increase the flexibility of my hamstrings to touch my toes within three months." SMART objective establish clear vision for success.

Designing a Balanced Chair Yoga Routine

1. Warm-up Exercises: Begin each session with gentle warm-up activities to prepare your body for more strenuous actions. Warm-up activities can include neck rolls, shoulder shrugs, and seated marches. These movements promote blood flow to the muscles and lessen the chance of damage.

2. Core Chair Yoga Poses: Incorporate a variety of chair yoga poses that address different parts of the body. Some basic poses include:

i. Seated Mountain Pose (Tadasana): Sit with your feet flat on the floor, spine straight, and hands resting on your thighs. This pose encourages strong posture and alignment.

ii. Seated Forward Bend (Paschimottanasana): Inhale and stretch your spine, then exhale and bend at the hips to fold forward, aiming for your toes or shins. This pose stretches the back and hamstrings.

iii. Seated Cat-Cow Stretch (Marjaryasana-Bitilasana): Alternate between arching your back (cow) and rounding your spine (cat) to mobilize the spine and reduce stress.

iv. Seated Spinal Twist(Ardha Matsyendrasana): Place your right hand on the back of the chair and your left hand on your right knee. Twist gently to the right, stretching your spine. Repeat on the other side. This pose helps with spinal flexibility and digestion.

v. Seated Pigeon Pose(Eka Pada Rajakapotasana): Cross your right ankle over your left knee and softly press down on your right knee. This position expands the hips and relieves stress in the lower back.

3. Breathwork and Relaxation: Incorporate breathwork (pranayama) and relaxation practices into your routine. Practices including deep diaphragmatic breathing, alternate nostril breathing, and guided relaxation help calm the mind and reduce stress.

4. Cool-down activities: End each session with easy cool-down activities to calm the body and mind. Cool-down exercises can include seated

forward bends, gentle twists, and deep breathing. These motions help convert the body from a state of activity to rest.

Monitoring Progress and Making Adjustments

1. Keeping a Practice Journal: Maintain a journal to chronicle your chair yoga practice. Record the activities you undertake, the duration of your sessions, and any remarks regarding your physical and mental state. A practice journal helps you track progress and discover areas for growth.

2. Regular self-assessment: Periodically examine your physical health, pain points, and progress toward your goals. Self-assessment lets you be aware of any changes in your body and alter your practice accordingly.

3. Adjusting the Routine: As you advance, gradually increase the intensity and duration of your practice. Introduce new positions and

variations to keep the workout interesting and enjoyable. Be conscious of your body's signals and avoid straining beyond your limitations to prevent injury.

4. Seeking Professional Guidance: Consider working with a trained chair yoga instructor, especially if you are new to yoga or have specific health problems. An instructor can provide personalized assistance, maintain appropriate alignment, and help you grow safely.

Sample Customized Chair Yoga Routine

Here is a sample chair yoga sequence that can be adapted based on individual requirements and capabilities:

1. Warm-up (5 minutes)
Neck rolls: 5 revolutions in each direction
Shoulder shrugs: 10 repetitions
Seated marches: march in place while seated for 1 minute.

2. Core Poses (20 minutes)

Seated Mountain Pose: Hold for 1 minute, focusing on breath and posture.

Seated Forward Bend: Hold for 5 breaths, repeat 2 times.

Seated Cat-Cow Stretch: 10 repetitions

Seated Spinal Twist: Hold for 5 breaths on each side, repeat 2 times.

Seated Pigeon Pose: Hold for 5 breaths on each side, repeat 2 times.

3. Breathwork and Relaxation (5 minutes): Diaphragmatic breathing: 10 deep breaths

Guided relaxation: Focus on relaxing each area of the body from head to toe.

4. Cool-down (5 minutes)

Seated Forward Bend: Hold for 5 breaths, repeat 2 times.

Gentle twists: Hold for 3 breaths on each side; repeat 2 times.

Developing a customized chair yoga training regimen entails a careful examination of personal requirements and capabilities, defining realistic and achievable goals, and ensuring safe progress over time. By analyzing your physical state, medical history, and personal preferences, you may design a tailored practice that matches your individual needs. Establishing a balanced regimen including warm-up exercises, core positions, breathwork, and relaxation techniques ensures a comprehensive approach to well-being. Regular monitoring and modifications, combined with professional assistance, help sustain a safe and productive practice. Embracing chair yoga can lead to greater flexibility, strength, stress reduction, and an overall enhanced quality of life.

Chapter 8

Including Chair Yoga in Everyday Activities

Chair yoga, a mild version of yoga performed while seated, is an easy way to integrate physical activity into daily routines. It offers several benefits, including enhanced flexibility, increased strength, and less stress. By introducing chair yoga into everyday tasks, you may smoothly integrate mindful movement into your life without the need for substantial time commitments or expensive equipment. This guide investigates ways to include chair yoga in brief morning and evening routines, while reading or watching TV, and through group sessions for socializing.

Quick Morning and Evening Routines

Starting and ending your day with chair yoga can establish a positive tone for the day and promote relaxation before bed. These brief exercises are designed to be efficient and effective, helping you to wake up energized and wind down comfortably.

Morning Routine

A morning chair yoga exercise should focus on mild stretches and motions to wake up the body and mind. Here's a suggested routine to start your day:

1. Seated Mountain Pose (Tadasana): Sit with your feet flat on the floor, spine straight, and hands resting on your thighs.
Close your eyes, take a few deep breaths, and establish an objective for the day.
Hold for 1 minute.

2.   Seated   Cat-Cow   Stretch (Marjaryasana-Bitilasana)
Place your hands on your knees.

Inhale, arch your back, and lift your chest (cow stance).
Exhale, curve your spine, and tuck your chin to your chest (cat stance).
Repeat for 5–10 breaths.

3. Seated Side Stretch: Raise your right arm overhead and rest your left hand on the chair for support.
Lean to the left, feeling a stretch down the right side of your body.
Hold for 5 breaths, then switch sides.

4. Seated Forward Bend (Paschimottanasana)
Inhale and stretch your spine.
Exhale, hinge at your hips, and fold forward, reaching toward your toes or shins.
Hold for 5–10 breaths.

5. Seated Spinal Twist (Ardha Matsyendrasana):
Place your right hand on the back of the chair and your left hand on your right knee.
Twist slowly to the right, stretching your spine.
Hold for 5 breaths, then switch sides.

Evening Routine

A nighttime chair yoga program should focus on relaxing and unwinding from the day's activities. Here's a sample regimen to help you prepare for a pleasant night's sleep:

1. Seated Neck Stretches: Bring your right ear to your right shoulder by gently tilting your head to the right.
After five breaths of holding, switch sides.
Proceed by gently tilting forward and backward.

2. Seated Shoulder Rolls: Lift your shoulders towards your ears, then roll them back and down.
Repeat for 5–10 revolutions.

3. Seated Forward Bend: Inhale and stretch your spine.
Exhale, hinge at your hips, and fold forward, reaching toward your toes or shins.
Hold for 5–10 breaths.

4. Seated Pigeon Pose (Eka Pada Rajakapotasana): Cross your right ankle over your left knee and softly press down on your right knee.
Hold for 5 breaths, then switch sides.

5. Seated Deep Breathing: Close your eyes and rest your hands on your tummy.
Take 10 deep, calm breaths, focusing on the rise and fall of your abdomen.

Chair Yoga While Reading or Watching TV

Incorporating chair yoga into activities like reading or watching TV can turn idle time into opportunities for mindful movement and stretching. These workouts are inconspicuous and can be completed without disrupting your activity.

Neck and Shoulder Stretches

1. Seated Neck Rolls: Slowly roll your head in a

circular manner.
Perform 5–10 revolutions in each direction.

2. Seated Shoulder Shrugs: Lift your shoulders towards your ears, hold for a moment, then release.
Repeat for 10 repetitions.

3. Seated Shoulder Blade Push: Sit up straight and push your shoulder blades together.
Hold for 5 seconds, then release.
Repeat for 10 repetitions.

Leg and Hip Stretches

1. Seated Leg Lifts: Extend your right leg out in front of you, keeping it straight.
Hold for a few seconds, then lower.
Repeat for 10 reps, then switch legs.

2. Seated Knee-to-Chest
Lift your right knee towards your chest and embrace it softly.
Hold for 5 breaths, then swap legs.

3. Seated Hip Circles: Place your feet flat on the floor and your hands on your hips.
Gently move your hips in a circular motion, performing 5–10 rotations in each direction.

Spine and Core Stretches

1. Seated Spinal Twist: Place your right hand on the back of the chair and your left hand on your right knee.
Twist slowly to the right, stretching your spine.
Hold for 5 breaths, then switch sides.

2. Seated Side Stretch: Raise your right arm overhead and rest your left hand on the chair for support.
Lean to the left, feeling a stretch down the right side of your body.
Hold for 5 breaths, then switch sides.

3. Seated Forward Bend: Inhale and stretch your spine.
Exhale, hinge at your hips, and fold forward,

reaching toward your toes or shins.
Hold for 5–10 breaths.

Chair Yoga Sessions in Groups and Socializing

Chair yoga may also be a social activity, allowing an opportunity to connect with others while engaging in a healthy practice. Group sessions can be planned in many settings, such as community centers, elder homes, businesses, or even at home with friends and family.

Benefits of Group Chair Yoga

1. Social Connection: Group chair yoga sessions create a sense of community and connection. Participants can share their experiences, support each other, and establish connections.
2. Motivation and Accountability: Practicing in a group can boost motivation and accountability. Regularly scheduled sessions provide a habit and encourage individuals to stay dedicated to their practice.

3. Guided Instruction: Group classes generally include a qualified instructor who may provide direction, maintain appropriate alignment, and adapt postures for varied abilities.

Organizing Group Chair Yoga Sessions

1. Choosing a Venue: Select a venue that is conveniently accessible and has enough space for participants to move comfortably. Community centers, retirement homes, and companies are great venues.

2. Scheduling Regular Sessions: Set a regular timetable for group sessions, such as once or twice a week. Consistency helps individuals incorporate chair yoga into their routines.

3. Hiring an Instructor: If possible, hire a professional chair yoga instructor to lead the sessions. They can provide professional coaching and ensure that exercises are completed safely.

4. Creating a friendly environment: Foster a friendly and inclusive climate where participants feel comfortable and supported. Encourage open

communication and feedback.

Sample Group Chair Yoga Session

Here's a sample format for a 30-minute group chair yoga session:

1. Introduction (5 minutes) Welcome everyone and introduce the session.
Briefly outline the benefits of chair yoga and the emphasis of the session.

2. Warm-up (5 minutes): Seated neck rolls: 5 rotations in each direction.
Seated shoulder shrugs: 10 repetitions.
Seated marches: march in place while seated for 1 minute.

3. Core Poses (15 minutes)
Seated Mountain Pose: Hold for 1 minute, focusing on breath and posture.
Seated Cat-Cow Stretch: 10 repetitions.
Seated Side Stretch: Hold for 5 breaths on each side.

Seated Spinal Twist: Hold for 5 breaths on each side.
Seated Forward Bend: Hold for 5–10 breaths.
Seated Pigeon Pose: Hold for 5 breaths on each side.

4. Breathwork and Relaxation (5 minutes): Diaphragmatic breathing: 10 deep breaths.
Guided relaxation: Focus on relaxing each portion of the body from head to toe.

5. Closing (5 minutes): Encourage participants to share their experiences or any feedback.
Provide strategies for implementing chair yoga into their daily lives.
Thank the attendees and remind them of the next session.

Tips for Socializing During Chair Yoga

1. Encourage Interaction: Create opportunities for participants to interact before and after the session. This can be fostered through icebreaker activities or discussion circles.

2. Celebrate successes: recognize and celebrate participants' successes, such as reaching a new stance or consistently attending sessions. This develops a sense of accomplishment and community.

3. Plan Social Events: Organize periodic social events outside of the chair yoga sessions, such as potlucks or group outings. These gatherings create social bonds and promote a sense of community.

Incorporating chair yoga into everyday tasks is a practical and efficient strategy to increase physical and mental well-being. By integrating fast morning and evening routines, doing chair yoga while reading or watching TV, and participating in group sessions, you may easily integrate mindful movement into your daily life. These techniques not only enhance flexibility, strength, and stress

Chapter 9

Case Studies and Success Stories

Chair yoga, a moderate form of yoga practiced while seated, has grown more popular among the elderly population due to its accessibility and multiple health benefits. This detailed guide analyzes various case studies and success stories of senior adults who have achieved considerable gains in their mobility and overall well-being via regular chair yoga practice.

Overview of Chair Yoga for Seniors

As people age, continuing physical activity becomes vital for sustaining mobility, strength, and independence. Traditional types of exercise can be problematic for many seniors due to limits in flexibility, balance, and strength. Chair yoga offers a potential answer, providing a low-impact, adaptive type of exercise that can be undertaken by people of varied fitness levels and physical capabilities.

Chair yoga involves modified yoga poses and stretches that can be done while seated or utilizing a chair for support. This practice emphasizes gentle movement, breathwork, and mindfulness, making it a good alternative for senior adults wishing to boost their physical and mental health.

Case Study 1: Margaret's Journey to Improved Flexibility

Background

Margaret, an 82-year-old retired schoolteacher, has been suffering stiffness and restricted range of motion in her joints owing to arthritis. She found it tough to accomplish daily activities like reaching for items on high shelves or bending down to pick up stuff from the floor. Margaret was looking for a form of exercise that could help increase her flexibility without inflicting additional pain or pressure on her joints.

Introduction to Chair Yoga

Margaret's daughter introduced her to chair yoga after attending a program at a nearby community center. Intrigued by the mild approach, Margaret decided to give it a try and joined a weekly chair yoga class specialized for seniors.

Progress and Results

Over the course of six months, Margaret regularly attended her chair yoga lessons and even tried some of the movements at home. The regimen includes easy stretches such as seated forward bends, seated spinal twists, and neck rolls, which helped to increase her flexibility and minimize stiffness.

Testimonial:

"Chair yoga has been a game-changer for me. I used to struggle with basic movements, but now

I can reach higher and bend lower without discomfort. The moderate stretches have relieved my arthritic discomfort and given me back some of my mobility. I feel more confident in my everyday duties and less dependent on others for help."

Conclusion

Margaret's story demonstrates how chair yoga may greatly increase flexibility and relieve the symptoms of arthritis in elderly adults. By adding regular practice, she was able to reclaim some of her independence and boost her quality of life.

Case Study 2: John's Path to Enhanced Balance and Stability

Background

John, a 75-year-old retired engineer, had been experiencing challenges with balance and stability, resulting in multiple falls over the past year. Concerned about his safety and freedom,

John sought an exercise regimen that could help him improve his balance and prevent future falls.

Introduction to Chair Yoga

John's physical therapist recommended chair yoga as a safe and effective technique to increase his balance and stability. John joined a local chair yoga class that concentrated on gentle strength-building exercises and balance positions.

Progress and Results

After three months of daily chair yoga practice, John noticed a substantial improvement in his balance and stability. The chair yoga practice featured exercises like seated leg lifts, seated marches, and modified tree poses, which helped strengthen his leg muscles and improve his coordination.

Testimonial:

"I was initially skeptical about chair yoga, but it has made a noticeable difference in my balance.

The exercises are gentle yet effective, and I've restored confidence in my ability to move around without fear of collapsing. Chair yoga has made me feel more stable and safe in my regular activities."

Conclusion

John's experience highlights the benefits of chair yoga in boosting balance and stability for elderly adults. Through constant practice, he was able to lower his risk of falling and improve his general sense of security and independence.

Case Study 3: Eleanor's Success in Alleviating Chronic Pain

Background

Eleanor, an 80-year-old grandmother, has been suffering from persistent lower back discomfort for several years. The pain hampered her movement and made it difficult for her to do hobbies she once loved, such as gardening and playing with her grandkids. Eleanor was looking for a gentle fitness routine that could help reduce her discomfort and enhance her quality of life.

Introduction to chair yoga

After attending a health session on the benefits of yoga for elders, Eleanor decided to try chair yoga. She enrolled in a class specifically developed for people with chronic pain and mobility difficulties.

Progress and Results

Over the next four months, Eleanor routinely attended her chair yoga classes, which included gentle stretches, seated twists, and deep breathing techniques. These movements helped to release tension in her lower back and improve her core muscles, ultimately lessening her persistent discomfort.

Testimonial:

"Chair yoga has been a blessing for me. The mild motions and stretches have improved my lower back pain tremendously. I can now spend more time in my garden and play with my grandchildren without difficulty. Chair yoga has improved my mobility and given me a new lease on life."

Conclusion

Eleanor's story highlights how chair yoga may be an excellent therapy for controlling and treating chronic pain in elderly adults. By adopting regular practice, she was able to lessen her pain and restore her ability to participate in things she enjoys.

Case Study 4: Robert's Improved Cardiovascular Health and Energy Levels

Background

Robert, a 78-year-old retired accountant, had been having poor energy levels and mild cardiovascular concerns. His doctor prescribed frequent exercise to help his heart health, but Robert found traditional forms of exercise too difficult. He was looking for a low-impact alternative that may enhance his energy levels and help his cardiovascular health.

Introduction to Chair Yoga

Robert discovered chair yoga through a senior wellness program at his local community center. He opted to take a class that concentrated on gentle aerobic motions and breathwork.

Progress and Results

After six months of daily chair yoga practice, Robert noticed an improvement in his energy levels and overall cardiovascular health. The practice included seated marches, seated sun salutations, and breathwork exercises that helped to boost his heart rate and enhance circulation.

Testimonial:

"Chair yoga has given me more energy and improved my heart health. The aerobic motions and breathwork are moderate yet effective, and I feel more bright and active. Chair yoga has been a wonderful addition to my daily regimen and has made me feel younger and more energetic."

Conclusion

Robert's experience demonstrates the benefits of chair yoga for improving cardiovascular health and enhancing energy levels in senior adults. Through constant practice, he was able to enhance his vigor and promote his entire well-being.

Case Study 5: Mary's Enhanced Mental and Emotional Well-Being

Background

Mary, an 83-year-old widow, had been feeling isolated and frightened since the demise of her husband. She struggled with loneliness and was looking for a means to better her mental and emotional well-being. Mary's daughter offered chair yoga as a potential option.

Introduction to Chair Yoga

Mary joined a chair yoga session at her local senior center that stressed mindfulness and relaxation. The social side of the class also appealed to her, giving her an opportunity to connect with others.

Progress and Results

Over several months, Mary routinely attended her chair yoga classes, which included mild stretches, breathing exercises, and guided meditation. These techniques helped to quiet her mind, reduce anxiety, and improve her emotional well-being. Additionally, the social connection with other class participants gave a sense of community and support.

Testimonial:

"Chair yoga has been a lifeline for me. The soothing motions and mindfulness activities have helped to calm my thoughts and ease my anxiety. I've also made new acquaintances in the class, which has helped me feel less alienated. Chair yoga has enhanced my mental and emotional well-being more than I could have imagined."

Conclusion

Mary's tale highlights the enormous influence chair yoga may have on mental and emotional well-being for senior folks. Through daily practice, she was able to minimize her anxiety, boost her mood, and discover a supportive community.

These case studies and success stories highlight the transformational impact of chair yoga for elderly people. Whether strengthening flexibility, enhancing balance and stability, reducing chronic pain, boosting cardiovascular health, or supporting mental and emotional well-being, chair yoga offers a gentle yet effective way for seniors to improve their quality of life. By introducing regular chair yoga practice into their routines, elderly individuals can realize considerable benefits in their mobility, independence, and overall health.

Conclusion

Chair yoga has emerged as a valuable and accessible type of exercise geared to fulfill the needs of seniors with restricted mobility. Its mild, adaptive nature makes it a wonderful choice for elders wishing to improve their mobility, health, and posture. This conclusion will highlight the important issues mentioned, stress the value of commencing chair yoga, and provide an incentive for senior folks to implement this practice into their daily lives.

Recap of Key Points

Accessibility and Safety

Chair yoga stands out owing to its accessibility. The use of a chair gives it stability, making it safe for those with varied degrees of movement. Unlike traditional yoga, which often requires getting up and down from the floor, chair yoga adapts poses to a seated position, thereby lowering the danger of falls and injuries. This function is vital for seniors who may have balance concerns or joint problems.

Enhanced Mobility

One of the most notable benefits of chair yoga is its potential to promote mobility. Through moderate stretches and motions, chair yoga helps increase joint flexibility and muscular strength. Regular practice can lead to an increased range of motion, making routine activities easier and more pleasant. Elderly adults who engage in chair yoga generally report being able to move more freely and with less pain, considerably increasing their quality of life.

Improved Health

Chair yoga adds to general wellness in various ways. It enhances cardiovascular health by slightly raising the heart rate and boosting circulation. The breathing exercises important to chair yoga promote respiratory function, making it simpler for senior adults to breathe deeply and efficiently. Additionally, the physical activity associated with chair yoga helps to maintain a healthy weight, reduce blood pressure, and enhance the immune system, contributing to a healthier lifestyle.

Better Posture

Good posture is vital for preventing musculoskeletal disorders and ensuring good body alignment. Chair yoga incorporates exercises that strengthen the core muscles and promote spinal alignment, hence improving posture. Elderly persons who practice chair yoga frequently generally find that their posture improves, lowering back discomfort and boosting comfort in daily tasks.

Mental and Emotional Benefits

Beyond physical wellness, chair yoga offers substantial mental and emotional advantages. The practice of mindfulness and relaxation practices can reduce stress, anxiety, and depression. Elderly individuals who participate in chair yoga generally enjoy a sense of tranquility and well-being, which boosts their overall quality of life. Additionally, chair yoga can create a sense of community, especially when performed in group settings, lessening feelings of isolation and loneliness.

Motivation for Starting Chair Yoga

Understanding the Need

As we age, being active becomes increasingly crucial for maintaining independence and quality of life. For senior adults with restricted mobility, finding a suitable kind of exercise can be tough. Chair yoga provides a practical alternative, delivering a low-impact, adaptive exercise choice that matches the special needs of seniors. Understanding the multiple benefits of chair yoga can drive individuals to give it a try.

Overcoming Barriers

Elderly persons may confront many challenges to establishing a new fitness practice, including physical, mental, and social obstacles. Chair yoga helps to overcome these barriers in numerous ways:

1. Physical Barriers: Chair yoga eliminates the need to get up and down from the floor, making it accessible for persons with physical restrictions. The use of a chair gives support and stability, lowering the danger of falls.

2. Mental Barriers: The soft nature of chair yoga makes it less scary than more intense kinds of exercise. Seniors can start with simple poses and gradually grow as their confidence and abilities improve.

3. Social Barriers: Chair yoga can be practiced alone or in groups, offering possibilities for social engagement. Group classes create a sense of community and support, encouraging regular participation.

Benefits Outweighing the Challenges

The benefits of chair yoga greatly exceed the challenges of establishing a new workout routine. Here are some convincing reasons to embrace chair yoga:

1. Ease of Practice: Chair yoga requires minimum space and no special equipment, making it easy to practice at home or in group settings.

2. Positive Reinforcement: Seeing modest improvements in mobility, strength, and posture can provide encouragement to continue practicing. The sensation of achievement and growth can increase confidence and self-esteem.

3. "Holistic Health": Chair yoga addresses both physical and mental health, delivering a holistic approach to well-being. The mix of physical activity, breathwork, and mindfulness promotes overall quality of life.

Advice and Adjustments for Starting Chair Yoga

Setting realistic goals

Setting realistic objective is key to sustainable motivation and measuring progress. Start with achievable short-term goals, such as practicing chair yoga for 10 minutes a day or perfecting a certain pose. Over time, create long-term goals, such as improving overall flexibility, lowering discomfort, or strengthening posture. Celebrate each progress to stay motivated and inspired.

Finding the Right Instructor or Program

Finding the correct instructor or program can make a major difference in the success of a chair yoga practice. Look for trained instructors who have experience working with older people. Many localities provide chair yoga programs specifically geared toward the elderly. Additionally, internet tools allow access to lectures and tutorials that may be practiced at home. Choose a program that meets your needs and comfort level.

Creating a Comfortable Practice Environment

Creating a comfortable and safe practice setting is vital for a great chair yoga experience. Ensure the practicing area is free from impediments and has a stable, comfy chair. Wear loose-fitting, comfortable clothes that allow for effortless movement. Establish a regular practice regimen to build consistency and make chair yoga a part of your daily routine.

Adapting Poses for Individual Needs

Adapting postures to individual requirements and limits is a crucial part of chair yoga. Use changes to make positions more accessible and comfortable. For example, use a cushion for added support or do poses at a slower tempo. Listen to your body and avoid any movements that create pain or discomfort. Gradually move to harder positions as your strength and flexibility increase.

Final Encouragement

Starting chair yoga can be a transformational experience for elderly adults with restricted mobility. The practice has several physical, mental, and emotional benefits, boosting the overall quality of life. By setting realistic goals, choosing the correct instructor or program, providing a comfortable practice environment, and customizing poses to individual needs, seniors can successfully incorporate chair yoga into their daily routines.

If you are an elderly senior trying to enhance your mobility, health, and posture, give chair yoga a try. Start with easy positions and progressively expand your practice. Remember, consistency is crucial. Over time, you will likely notice considerable gains in your physical capabilities and overall well-being. Chair yoga can be a wonderful addition to your daily routine, helping you to enjoy a more active, healthy, and satisfying life.

Chair yoga is more than just a type of exercise; it is a gateway to enhanced mobility, improved health, and better posture. By embracing chair yoga, older adults with restricted mobility can access a world of benefits that contribute to a healthier, more vibrant existence. Start today and take the first step towards a more active and fulfilling future.